# ANTI-INFLAM

# DIET COOKBOOK
## *FOR BEGINNERS*

**A Simple Guide to Kickstart Your Wellness Journey with Delicious Anti-inflammatory Recipes**

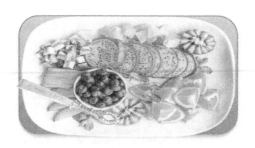

## CHERYL C. SMITH

**GET ACCESS TO MORE OF MY BOOK**

**2 Anti-Inflammatory Diet Cookbook for Beginners**

# TABLE OF CONTENTS

# INTRODUCTION

Walter, an elderly man living in the lovely community of Harmony Springs, was plagued by a constant discomfort in his joints. In search of peace, he came across the concept of an anti-inflammatory diet.

Walter was intrigued, so he changed his eating habits, substituting colorful veggies, lean proteins, and antiinflammatory spices for processed foods. The rigidity in his joints gradually faded, and the continuous ache became a mere murmur.

A gradual transition occurred when Walter embraced this gastronomic shift. His energy levels increased, and he rediscovered joy in previously forgotten pastimes. The townspeople admired the revitalized Walter, attributing his increased vitality to the power of a well-balanced diet.

Walter's quest became a whispered story of inspiration that echoed across Harmony Springs. His narrative demonstrated the transforming power of adopting a better lifestyle, demonstrating that aging might be defied via attentive eating. The perfume of anti-inflammatory spices lingered in the heart of town, a tribute to the incredible journey of an old man who regained life through the foods on his plate.

# Understanding Inflammation

Inflammation is the body's natural response to damage or infection. For example, if you cut your finger, the area around the wound will become red, swollen, and painful. This is due to the fact that your body is sending white blood cells and other immune cells to the location to combat infection and repair the wound.

**Inflammation is classified into two types:** acute and chronic. Acute inflammation is usually temporary and fades within a few weeks. In contrast, chronic inflammation can linger for months or even years.

## Acute inflammation:

Acute inflammation is a natural and healthy reaction to an injury or infection. It aids in the protection of the body and the healing of damaged tissue. Acute inflammation symptoms can include:

* Redness
* Swelling
* Pain
* Warmth
* Function Loss

Acute inflammation usually resolves on its own. However, if it is severe or does not resolve itself, it can cause difficulties.

## Chronic inflammation:

Chronic inflammation is a long-term disorder that can cause tissue and organ damage.
Chronic inflammation symptoms can range from moderate to severe. They may include the following:

* Fatigue
* Muscle ache
* Joint pain
* Skin rash
* Fever

You can reduce inflammation and promote general health and well-being by embracing this dietary cookbook.

## Importance of Anti-Inflammatory Diet

The importance of an anti-inflammatory diet derives from its ability to improve health.
Some important reasons are:

**Reduces Chronic Inflammation**: Reduces chronic inflammation, lowering the risk of diseases such as heart disease and diabetes.

**Supports Joint Health**: Promotes joint health and relieves symptoms associated with illnesses such as arthritis.

**Maintains Blood Sugar Levels**: Complex carbohydrates, fiber, and healthy fats help to keep blood sugar levels constant.

**Heart Health:** Improves lipid profiles and reduces inflammation to support cardiovascular health.

**Aids Digestive Health**: Promotes digestive well-being by contributing to a healthy gut, lowering inflammation, and boosting digestive well-being.

**Weight Management:** Promotes balanced, nutrient-dense diets to aid with weight management.

**Improves Immune Function**: Provides important nutrients for a strong immune system, improving the body's ability to fight infections.

**Promotes Overall Well-Being**: By nourishing the body and mind, it improves energy levels, mood, and overall sense of well-being.

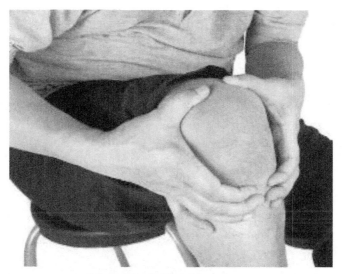

**Chronic Inflammation**

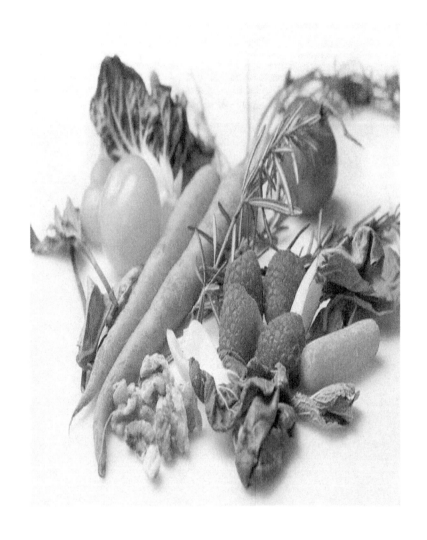

# VEGETABLE FRUITES

## 10 Anti-Inflammatory Diet Cookbook for Beginners

# CHAPTER 1: BASICS OF ANTIINFLAMMATORY EATING

An anti-inflammatory diet, which includes plenty of fruits, vegetables, and whole grains while minimizing processed foods, red meat, and sugary drinks, can help reduce inflammation.

## What is an Anti-Inflammatory Diet?

An anti-inflammatory diet is a diet that focuses on lowering inflammation in the body. It usually includes a lot of fruits, vegetables, and whole grains, while avoiding processed foods, red meat, and sugary drinks.

## Key Principles and Guidelines

The following are the main principles and recommendations to follow:

### Make whole, unprocessed foods a priority:

- *Fruits and vegetables*: Aim for at least 5 servings of a rainbow per day. They are high in antioxidants and fiber, both of which are important for decreasing inflammation.

- *Whole Grains*: For fiber and complex carbs that help manage blood sugar levels, choose brown rice, quinoa, whole-wheat bread, and oats.

- *Healthy fats*: Anti-inflammatory sources of healthy fats include olive oil, avocado, almonds, and seeds.

- *Lean Protein Sources:* For critical nutrients without inflammatory saturated fats, choose fish, chicken, lentils, and beans.

## Reduce intake of processed foods:

- *Fast food and package meals:* these are heavy in unhealthy fats, salt, refined sugars, and artificial additives, which all lead to inflammation.

- *Processed Meats*: Limit sausages, bacon, deli meats and hot dogs, because they have been associated with higher inflammation indicators.

- **Sugary Drinks and Refined Sugars**: To avoid blood sugar spikes and inflammation, avoid sodas, juices, and sugary snacks.

## Make Use of Anti-Inflammatory Spices:

- **Turmeric**: Curcumin, the main ingredient in turmeric, has significant anti-inflammatory actions.

- **Ginger**: Ginger is well-known for its ability to relieve nausea and pain, but it also has anti-inflammatory properties.

- **Garlic**: This multipurpose herb contains antiinflammatory antioxidants and sulfur compounds.

- **Cinnamon**: Aids in blood sugar regulation and has anti-inflammatory qualities.

## Use Caution When Choosing Cooking Methods:

- **Grilling, broiling, baking, and steaming:** When compared to frying, these procedures reduce the development of inflammatory chemicals.

- **Reduce deep frying and high-heat cooking**:

Avoid techniques that produce advanced glycation end products (AGEs), which have been related to inflammation and chronic illnesses.

## Consider Gut Health:

- *Probiotics*: Fermented foods such as yogurt, kimchi, and sauerkraut contain beneficial bacteria that aid in gut health and inflammation reduction.

- *Prebiotics*: Foods like bananas, onions, and asparagus promote a healthy microbiome by feeding the good gut bacteria.

## Maintain Hydration:

- Drinking plenty of water aids in the removal of pollutants and promotes overall health, including the reduction of inflammation.

## Personalize Your Approach:

- When creating an anti-inflammatory diet plan, consider your health circumstances, food allergies, and preferences.
- For personalized advice, speak with a healthcare practitioner or a licensed dietitian.

## Make Long-Term Changes:

- Begin by adding tiny modifications gradually to make the transition to anti-inflammatory eating sustainable and enjoyable.
- For long-term success, focus on developing healthy habits rather than tight limitations.

You may embrace the benefits of an anti-inflammatory diet and live a happier, more vibrant life by following these ideas and practices. Remember that consistency and a balanced approach are essential for optimizing the benefits of this nutritional regimen.

# Foods to Include and Avoid

## Foods to include:

**Fruits**: Fruits include antioxidants, which can aid in reducing inflammation. Try to consume five or more servings of fruits and vegetables each day.

**Vegetables:** Vegetables are high in antioxidants and fiber, both of which can aid to reduce inflammation. Try to consume at least five servings of vegetables per day.

**Whole grains:** Whole grains are high in fiber, which can aid in the reduction of inflammation. Instead of white bread, white rice, and pasta, choose whole-wheat bread, brown rice, and quinoa.

**Healthy fats:** Healthy fats such as olive oil, avocados, and almonds can aid in inflammation reduction.

**Spices:** Spices such as turmeric, ginger, and cinnamon can also aid in inflammation reduction.

## Foods to avoid:

**Processed foods**: Processed foods are frequently heavy in harmful fats, sugar, and salt, all of which can lead to inflammation.

**Red meat**: While red meat is high in protein, it can also lead to inflammation. Consume red meat in moderation or select lean cuts.

*Sugary beverages*: Sugary drinks include a lot of added sugar, which can cause inflammation. Instead, drink water, unsweetened tea, or coffee.

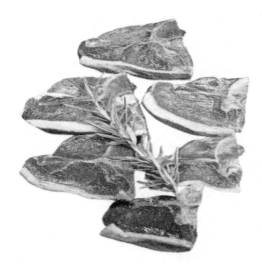

## AVOID RED MEAT

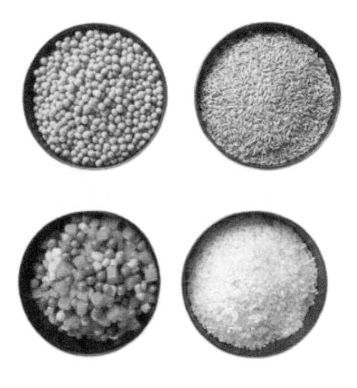

## WHOLE GRAINS

18 Anti-Inflammatory Diet Cookbook for Beginners

# CHAPTER 2: BUILDING YOUR ANTI-INFLAMMATORY KITCHEN

## Stocking Essential Ingredients

Stocking your cupboard and fridge with anti-inflammatory foods is the first step in creating an anti-inflammatory kitchen. Concentrate on fresh, complete meals high in antioxidants, fiber, and healthy fats, while avoiding processed foods and inflammatory factors. Here's a list of necessary ingredients:

## Pantry Essentials:

- *Whole Grains*: Brown rice, quinoa, oats, wholewheat pasta, barley, and so on.
- *Beans and legumes*: lentils, chickpeas, black beans, kidney beans, and others.
- **Nuts and seeds:** chia seeds, walnuts, Almonds, flaxseeds, pumpkin seeds, etc.
- *Spices*: turmeric, ginger, garlic, cinnamon, cumin, coriander, oregano, and others.
- *Dried herbs*: thyme, basil, rosemary, parsley, and others.
- *Oils:* olive oil, avocado oil, flaxseed oil
- *Vinegars:* Balsamic vinegar and apple cider vinegar

**19 Anti-Inflammatory Diet Cookbook for Beginners**

- **Natural sweeteners:** honey or maple syrup • **Tea:** Green tea, ginger tea, chamomile tea, etc.

## Fridge Staples:

- **Fruits**: Berries, apples, bananas, citrus fruits, and so on.
- **Vegetables**: leafy greens, broccoli, carrots, bell peppers, onions, and so on.
- **Lean protein**: chicken, fish, tofu, tempeh, and so on.
- **Eggs**: A diverse source of protein and good fats.
- **Dairy substitutes**: unsweetened almond milk, yogurt, and kefir (if tolerated).
- **Fermented foods** (optional): kimchi, sauerkraut, kombucha, etc.

## Additional Suggestions:

- Whenever possible, get organic produce.
- Buy in bulk to save money and cut down on packing waste.
- In a windowsill garden, you can grow your own herbs.
- To avoid impulse purchases, plan your meals and create a grocery list.

- To extend the shelf life of ingredients, store them appropriately.

# Cooking Tools and Techniques

You can unlock the full potential of anti-inflammatory cooking if you have the correct equipment and practices. Consider the following basic tools and techniques:

## Essential Tools:
- A cutting board and a good quality knife
- A blender or food processor
- A steamer
- A cast iron skillet or a barbecue pan
- Baking pans
- Cups and spoons for measuring
- Containers for storage **Cooking Methods:**

- *Grilling and roasting*: reduce fat intake while providing taste and texture.
- *Steaming and boiling*: are gentle cooking methods that keep nutrients intact.
- *Sautéing and stir-frying:* To avoid burning, use healthy oils and short cooking periods.
- *Baking and roasting*: are excellent methods for cooking vegetables and lean protein sources.

## Additional Suggestions:

- For flavor, use less salt and experiment with herbs and spices.
- Select methods that use as little oil as possible, such as baking and steaming.
- Read recipes carefully and adhere to cooking times and temperatures specified.
- Experiment with various flavors and ingredients to create recipes that you like.
- Don't be afraid to experiment in the kitchen!

You can produce tasty anti-inflammatory meals at home by filling your kitchen with key items and learning basic culinary methods. Remember that the key to obtaining the advantages of anti-inflammatory nutrition is to consume fresh, complete foods and use healthy cooking methods.

# CHAPTER 3: BREAKFAST RECIPES

Start your day off right with these anti-inflammatory breakfast recipes:

## Energizing Smoothie Bowls

Smoothie bowls are a quick, easy, and nutritious way to start the day. They're high in fruits, veggies, healthy fats, and protein, making them a nutritious and filling breakfast option.

**Ingredients:**
- 1 cup frozen berries
- 1 frozen or fresh banana
- 1/2 cup kale or spinach
- 1/2 light almond or coconut milk
- 1/4 avocado
- 1 scoop protein powder (optional)
- Toppings of choice: granola, almonds, seeds, chia seeds, fresh fruit slices etc.

**Instructions:**

- Blend everything but the toppings until smooth and creamy.
- Pour the smoothie into a bowl and garnish with your preferred toppings.

**Tips:**
- Experiment with various fruits and veggies to discover your favorite combinations.
- For a more filling smoothie, add protein powder.
- To add healthful fats, use nut butter or ground flaxseeds.
- For an added taste boost, top your smoothie bowl with fresh herbs.

# Quinoa Breakfast Porridge

This hearty and filling porridge is a tasty spin on conventional oats. It's high in protein, fiber, and minerals, so you'll feel full and energized all morning.

## Ingredients:
- 1/2 cup washed dry quinoa
- 1 cup unsweetened almond or coconut milk.
- 1 cup of water
- 1/4 teaspoon cinnamon powder
- 1 tsp. nutmeg

- 1/4 cup chopped nuts or seeds
- 1/4 cup chopped fresh fruit
- Optional: honey or maple syrup to taste

## Instructions:
- Combine the quinoa, almond milk, water, cinnamon, and nutmeg in a medium saucepan.

- Bring to a boil, then reduce to a low heat and continue to cook for 15-20 minutes, or until the quinoa is fluffy and cooked through.
- Heat for another minute after adding the nuts and seeds.
- Remove from heat and, if preferred, whisk in honey or maple syrup.
- Serve warm with fresh fruit on top.

## Tips:
- Add a tablespoon of shredded coconut or nut butter to the porridge for a deeper flavor.
- To provide variety, use a variety of nuts and seeds.
- Try various spices, such as ginger or cardamom.
- For a more filling breakfast, add a scoop of protein powder.

# Turmeric Scrambled Eggs

Scrambled eggs are a traditional breakfast item, and the addition of turmeric gives them a brilliant color as well as an anti-inflammatory benefit. This meal is quick to prepare and high in protein and healthy fats.

## Ingredients:
- 2 eggs
- 1 teaspoon of coconut oil
- 1/4 teaspoon turmeric powder
- 1/4 teaspoon cumin powder
- 1 tsp salt and pepper
- Optional toppings: diced avocado, fresh herbs, salsa, etc.

## Instructions:
- In a mixing bowl, combine the eggs, coconut oil, turmeric, cumin, salt, and pepper.
- Melt butter in a nonstick skillet over medium heat.
- Pour in the egg mixture and cook, stirring regularly, until the eggs are scrambled to your liking.
- Serve immediately with your preferred garnishes.

## Tips:
- To make the eggs smoother, add a dash of milk or cream.

- To add more nutrients and flavor, add chopped veggies such as spinach or bell peppers.
- Add nutritional yeast for cheesy flavor and additional protein.
- Serve your scrambled eggs with whole-wheat bread or with a side of fruit.

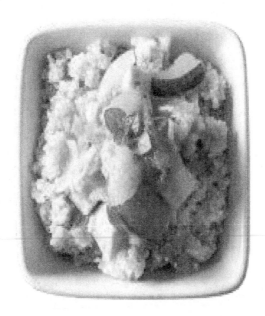

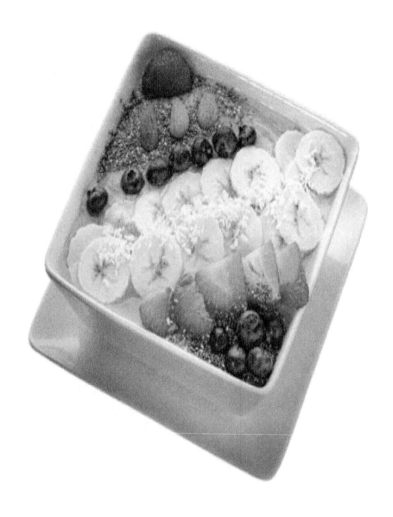

**SMOOTHIE FRUIT BOWL**

**28 Anti-Inflammatory Diet Cookbook for Beginners**

# CHAPTER 4: LUNCH AND DINNER IDEAS

## Avocado Salsa with Grilled Salmon

This light and delicious summer dish is ideal for lunch or dinner. The salmon contains protein and omega-3 fatty acids, and the avocado salsa adds taste and healthful lipids.

### Ingredients:
- 2 fillets of salmon
- 1 tablespoon extra-virgin olive oil
- pepper and salt to taste
- 1 chopped ripe avocado
- 1/2 cup red onion, chopped
- 1/4 cup cilantro, chopped
- 1 juiced lime
- Optional garnishes: chopped fresh herbs, crumbled feta cheese, and so on.

### Instructions:

**29 Anti-Inflammatory Diet Cookbook for Beginners**

- 
  Heat the grill or grill pan to medium-high.
- Use salt and pepper to season the salmon fillets.
- Grill the salmon for 4-5 minutes per side, or until done.
- Meanwhile, in a mixing dish, combine the avocado, red onion, cilantro, and lime juice.
- Serve grilled salmon with avocado salsa and desired garnishes.

**Tips:**

- Add a sprinkle of smoked paprika to the avocado salsa for a smokey taste.
- Replace salmon with other types of fish, such as trout or cod.
- Serve the grilled salmon with roasted veggies or quinoa on the side.

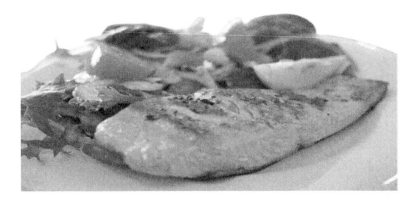

# Chickpea and Spinach Stew

This filling and tasty stew is high in protein, fiber, and minerals. It's a hearty and filling dish that's ideal for a cold winter day.

## Ingredients:
- 1 tablespoon extra virgin olive oil
- 1 diced onion
- 2 minced garlic cloves
- 1 teaspoon cumin powder
- 1 tablespoon turmeric powder
- Optional: a pinch of chili flakes
- 1 cup diced tomatoes
- 1 can (15 oz) washed and drained chickpeas • 4 cups vegetable broth
- 4 cups fresh spinach, chopped • pepper and salt to taste.
- Optional garnishes include chopped fresh herbs, lemon wedges, etc.

## Instructions:
- Heat the olive oil in a big pot or Dutch oven over medium heat.
- Cook until the onion is softened, about 5 minutes.
- Cook for another minute, or until the garlic, cumin, turmeric, and chili flakes (if using) are aromatic.

- 
- 
  Cook until the tomatoes have softened and released their juices, about 5 minutes.
  Stir in the chickpeas, vegetable broth, and spinach. Bring to a boil, then reduce to a low heat and continue to cook for 15 minutes, or until the veggies are soft.
- Season to taste with salt and pepper.
- Serve immediately with your preferred toppings.

**Tips:**
- For more nutrients and taste, add a can of diced sweet potatoes or carrots to the stew.
- For a deeper flavor, use vegetable broth instead of water.
- Serve the stew with whole-grain bread or brown rice on the side.

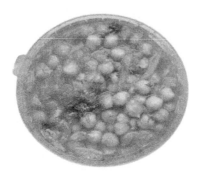

# Vegetarian Stir-Fry

This vibrant and fragrant stir-fry is a quick and easy way to get your daily vegetable intake. It's high in vitamins, minerals, and fiber, and it's ready in less than 30 minutes.

## Ingredients:
- 1 tablespoon extra virgin olive oil
- 1 sliced onion
- 1 sliced bell pepper
- 1 cup florets broccoli
- 1/2 cup carrots, chopped
- 1/2 cup mushrooms, chopped
- 1 tablespoon soy sauce
- 1 tbsp honey (or maple syrup)
- 1 tbsp Sriracha sauce (optional)
- 1 cup brown rice or quinoa, cooked
- 1 cup fresh kale or spinach

## Instructions:
- In a large wok or skillet, heat the olive oil over medium-high heat.
- Combine the onion, bell pepper, broccoli, carrots, and mushrooms in a mixing bowl.
- The vegetables should be stir-fried for 5 to 7 minutes, or until they are crisp-tender.

- 

- 
  In a small bowl, combine the soy sauce, honey, and sriracha (if using).
  Stir in the sauce and cook for another minute with the vegetables.
- Stir in cooked brown rice or quinoa until heated through.
- Cook until the spinach or kale has wilted.
- Serve right away.

**Tips:**

- Use other veggies, such as zucchini, snap peas, or bok choy.
- For extra protein, add a tofu scramble or tempeh.
- Serve the stir-fry with brown rice or noodles on the side.

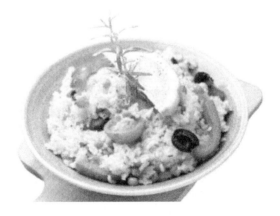

## Nut and Seed Trail Mix

This is a traditional snack that is both nutritious and filling. It's high in protein, healthy fats, and fiber, making it ideal for a quick energy boost in between meals.

### Ingredients:
- 1 cup uncooked almonds
- 1/2 cup walnuts
- 1/4 cup pumpkin seeds
- 1/4 cup sunflower seeds
- 1/4 cup dried cranberries
- 1/4 cup shredded unsweetened coconut
- Optional: 1/4 cup dark chocolate chips

### Instructions:
- Toss all of the ingredients together in a mixing basin.
- Refrigerate in an airtight container for up to one week.

### Tips:
To find your preferred mix, try different nuts, seeds, and dried fruits.

For added taste, sprinkle with cinnamon or sea salt.

- 

- 

- Add a scoop of protein powder to the mix for a more satisfying snack.

# Roasted Red Pepper Hummus

This bright and delicious hummus is ideal for dipping vegetables or pita bread in. It's a tasty and nutritious snack high in protein, fiber, and healthy fats.

**Ingredients:**
- 1 can (15 oz) washed and drained chickpeas
- 1 peeled and seeded roasted red pepper
- 1 tbsp tahini
- 2 tbsp of olive oil
- 2 tbsp of lemon juice
- 1 minced garlic clove
- 1/2 teaspoon cumin powder
- 1/4 teaspoon salt
- Optional: a pinch of cayenne pepper
- water as needed

**Instructions:**
- In a food processor, combine all of the ingredients and blend until smooth, adding water as needed to obtain the desired consistency.

- With fresh vegetables, pita bread, or crackers, serve.

**Tips:**
- For a smokier flavor, roast your own red peppers.
- Other roasted vegetables, such as beets or carrots, can be added to the hummus to add taste and nutrients.
- Try other herbs and spices, such as smoked paprika or coriander.

# Cucumber Avocado Bites

These light and nutritious nibbles are ideal for a snack or appetizer. They are high in vitamins, minerals, and good fats, making them a filling and nutritious option.

**Ingredients:**
- 1 cucumber (cut into rounds)
- 1 peeled and thinly sliced avocado
- 1 tablespoon feta cheese, crumbled
- 1/4 cup fresh cilantro, chopped
- 1 tablespoon lime juice

- 

pepper and salt to taste

**Instructions:**
- On a platter, arrange cucumber slices.
- Add avocado slices, feta cheese, cilantro, lime juice, salt, and pepper to each cucumber slice.
- Serve right away.

**Tips:**
- For perfectly thin cucumber slices, use a mandoline slicer.
- For a spicy boost, add a squeeze of sriracha or crushed red pepper flakes.
- Drizzle with balsamic glaze to add sweetness.

Remember that the goal is to choose fresh, whole foods and to prepare them in simple, nutritious ways.

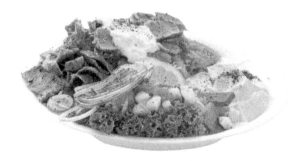

## Kale and Quinoa Salad

This colorful and tasty salad is high in minerals and protein. It makes an excellent side dish for any dinner and is high in vitamins, minerals, and fiber.

**Ingredients:**
- 2 cups kale, chopped
- 1 cup cooked quinoa
- 1/2 cup minced red onion
- 1/4 cup chopped dried cranberries
- 1/4 cup walnuts, chopped
- 1/4 cup feta cheese, crumbled

**For the dressing:** •
3 tbsp olive oil
- 2 tbsp of lemon juice
- 1 tbsp honey (or maple syrup) • 1 tablespoon Dijon mustard • salt and pepper to taste.

**Instructions:**
- Combine the kale, quinoa, red onion, cranberries, walnuts, and feta cheese in a large mixing basin.

- 

  Whisk together the olive oil, lemon juice, honey, Dijon mustard, salt, and pepper in a separate bowl.
- Toss the salad with the dressing to coat.
- Serve right away.

**Tips:**

- To tenderize the kale, massage it with a little olive oil before adding the other ingredients.
- Other chopped veggies, such as carrots or bell peppers, can be added to the salad for extra taste and benefits.
- For a vegan version, substitute avocado slices for the feta cheese.

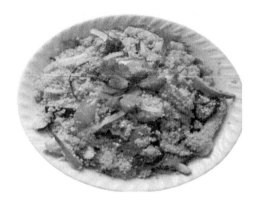

# Roasted Sweet Potato Wedges

Sweet potato wedges are a more wholesome substitute for French fries. They're high in vitamins, fiber, and antioxidants, making them a filling and healthy side dish.

## Ingredients:
- 2 big sweet potatoes, peeled and cut into wedges
- 1 tablespoon extra-virgin olive oil
- 1 teaspoon of sea salt
- 1/4 teaspoon ground black pepper
- Optional spices: garlic powder, paprika, and cumin.

## Instructions:
- Preheat the oven to 425°F/220°C.
- Using parchment paper, line a baking sheet.
- Toss sweet potato wedges with olive oil, salt, pepper, and any additional spices to taste.
- Arrange the wedges on the baking sheet in a single layer.
- Bake for 20-25 minutes, or until crispy and tender, flipping halfway through.
- Quickly serve with your preferred dipping sauce.

**Tips**:

- 

- To ensure equal cooking, cut the sweet potatoes into regular wedges.
  To crisp up the sweet potato wedges, soak them in water for 15 minutes before roasting.
- Experiment with various spices and herbs to add flavor.

## Citrusy Broccoli Slaw

This vivid and refreshing slaw is a fantastic way to get more vegetables into your diet. It's high in vitamins, minerals, and fiber, making it a nutritious and filling side dish.

### Ingredients:

- 2 cups broccoli, shredded
- 1 cup carrots, shredded
- 1/2 cup red onion, chopped • 1/4 cup fresh cilantro, chopped • To make the dressing:
- 2 tbsp of olive oil
- two tbsp orange juice
- 1 tbsp honey (or maple syrup)
- 1 tablespoon vinegar (rice)
- 1 tsp. grated orange zest

- Season to taste with salt and pepper.

## Instructions:

- Combine broccoli, carrots, red onion, and cilantro in a large mixing bowl.
- Whisk together the olive oil, orange juice, honey, rice vinegar, orange zest, salt, and pepper in a separate bowl.
- Toss the slaw with the dressing to coat.
- Serve right away.

## Tips:

- To make preparation easier, shred the vegetables in a food processor.
- Other chopped vegetables, such as bell peppers or cabbage, can be added to the slaw to add taste and nutrients.
- For a different zesty flavor, substitute lime juice for orange juice.

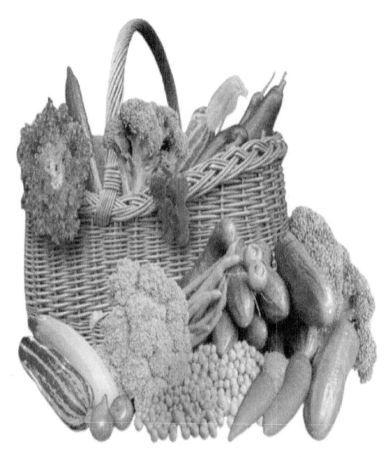

**VEGETABLES**

**44 Anti-Inflammatory Diet Cookbook for Beginners**

# CHAPTER 7: DESSERTS WITH A TWIST

With these tasty and anti-inflammatory sweets, you may satisfy your sweet desire without jeopardizing your health:

## Berry Chia Seed Pudding

Protein, fiber, and antioxidants are abundant in this creamy and delicious pudding. It's a quick and easy dessert that's ideal for a hot summer day.

### Ingredients:
- 1 chia seed cup
- 1 cup almond or coconut milk, unsweetened
- 1 tablespoon honey or maple syrup
- 1 tsp vanilla extract
- 1/4 cup berries, mixed
- Optional toppings: more berries, granola, and coconut flakes

### Instructions:
- Combine chia seeds, almond milk, honey, and vanilla essence in a container or bowl.

- Allow for at least 30 minutes, or until the chia seeds have absorbed the liquid and formed a thick pudding.
- In a serving glass, layer the pudding with the mixed berries.
- Choose your own additional toppings.
- Allow at least 2 hours before serving to chill.

**Tips:**
- To add variety, use different varieties of berries or other fruits.
- For more protein, add a scoop of protein powder to the pudding.
- Use full-fat coconut milk for a more pronounced flavor.

# Dark Chocolate Avocado Mousse

This luscious and creamy mousse is high in antioxidants, fiber, and healthy fats. It's a guilt-free treat that's ideal for a special occasion.

**Ingredients:**
- 2 peeled and pitted ripe avocados
- 1/2 cup chocolate powder, unsweetened
- 1 tablespoon honey or maple syrup

- 1 tbsp. vanilla extract
- 1/4 cup milk (dairy or nondairy)
- 1 teaspoon salt

## Instructions:
- Blend avocados, cocoa powder, honey, vanilla essence, milk, and salt in a food processor until smooth and creamy.
- Adjust the sweetness or cocoa powder to taste.
- Divide the mousse among serving glasses and place in the refrigerator for at least 2 hours before serving.

## Tips:
- For the best texture, use ripe avocados.
- For a spicy kick, add a pinch of cayenne pepper.
- For added taste and texture, top the mousse with fresh berries or chopped almonds.

# Ginger Turmeric Golden Milk Popsicles

These pleasant and healthful popsicles are high in antiinflammatory compounds and taste fantastic. On a hot day, they're ideal for a nutritious and filling snack.

## Ingredients:

- 2 cups almond or coconut milk, unsweetened
- 1 teaspoon turmeric powder
- 1/4 cup ginger, grated
- 1 tablespoon honey or maple syrup
- 1 tsp vanilla extract
- a pinch of cinnamon
- a pinch of black pepper

## Instructions:

- Warm almond milk or coconut milk with turmeric powder and ginger in a saucepan.
- Cook for 5 minutes, stirring occasionally, at a low heat.
- Remove the ginger by straining the mixture.
- Stir in the honey, vanilla essence, cinnamon, and black pepper to the filtered liquid.
- Freeze the mixture in popsicle molds for at least 4 hours, or until the mixture is solid.

## Tips:

- For the finest flavor, use fresh ginger.
- For a spicy kick, add a pinch of cayenne pepper.
- Replace cinnamon with other spices such as cardamom or nutmeg.

# 30-Day Anti-Inflammatory Meal Plan for Beginners

This diet includes anti-inflammatory breakfast, lunch, supper, and snack alternatives for each day. Remember to modify the portions as necessary.

## Week 1

### Day 1:

**breakfast***:* Oatmeal with berries and cinnamon.
**Lunch***:* leftover chicken stir-fry with vegetables and brown rice.
**Dinner***:* Roasted salmon with quinoa and roasted vegetables.
Snack: Fruit salad with yogurt.

### Day 2:

**Breakfast***:* Scrambled eggs with spinach and tomatoes.
**Lunch***:* Lentil soup with whole-grain bread.
**49 Anti-Inflammatory Diet Cookbook for Beginners**

**Dinner***:* brown rice and stir-fried tofu with veggies.
**Snack***:* Hummus and vegetables.

## Day 3:

**Breakfast***:* Chia seed pudding with fruit and almonds.
**Lunch***:* Black bean burgers on whole-wheat buns with avocado and salsa.
**Dinner***:* Turkey chili with whole-wheat bread.
**Snack***:* Nuts and seeds

## Day 4:

**Breakfast:** Smoothie with spinach, banana, mango, and yogurt
**Lunch:** Salmon salad with quinoa and avocado
**Dinner:** Lentil soup with whole-grain bread
**Snack:** Hard-boiled eggs

## Day 5:

**Breakfast:** Greek yogurt with berries and chia seeds
**Lunch***:* Brown rice and vegetables stir-fried with chicken
**Dinner**: Roasted chicken with roasted vegetables **Snack:** Trail mix

### Day 6:

**Breakfast**: Scrambled eggs with spinach and tomatoes
**Lunch**: Leftover tofu stir-fry with vegetables and brown rice
**Dinner**: Salmon with quinoa and roasted vegetables
**Snack**: Fruit salad with yogurt

### Day 7:

**Breakfast**: Chia seed pudding with fruit and nuts **Lunch**: Black bean burgers on whole-wheat buns with avocado and salsa
**Dinner**: Turkey chili with whole-wheat bread
**Snack**: Nuts and seeds

## Week 2

### Day 8:

**Breakfast**: Smoothie with spinach, banana, mango, and yogurt
**Lunch**: Salmon salad with quinoa and avocado
**Dinner**: Lentil soup with whole-grain bread
**Snack**: Hard-boiled eggs

**51 Anti-Inflammatory Diet Cookbook for Beginners**

## Day 9:

**Breakfast**: Greek yogurt with berries and chia seeds
**Lunch**: Brown rice and vegetables stir-fried with chicken
**Dinner**: Roasted chicken with roasted vegetables
**Snack**: Trail mix

## Day 10:

**Breakfast**: Scrambled eggs with spinach and tomatoes
**Lunch**: Leftover salmon with quinoa and roasted vegetables
**Dinner**: Salmon with quinoa and roasted vegetables
**Snack**: Fruit salad with yogurt

## Day 11:

*Breakfast:* Overnight oats with berries and nuts
**Lunch**: Tuna salad with whole-wheat crackers and vegetables
**Dinner**: Sweet potato baked with avocado and black beans **Snack**: Edamame

## Day 12:

**Breakfast**: Smoothie with spinach, pineapple, ginger, and almond milk
**Lunch**: Leftover baked sweet potato with black beans and avocado
**Dinner**: Turkey burgers on whole-wheat buns with grilled vegetables
**Snack**: Greek yogurt with granola and honey

## Day 13:

**Breakfast**: Chia seed pudding with coconut milk and mangoes
**Lunch**: Chicken Caesar salad with whole-grain bread
**Dinner**: Vegetarian chili with cornbread
**Snack**: Cottage cheese with berries and chia seeds

## Day 14:

**Breakfast**: Scrambled eggs with smoked salmon and spinach
**Lunch**: grilled chicken and veggies on quinoa salad
**Dinner**: Salmon with roasted asparagus and quinoa
**Snack**: Dark chocolate and almonds

# Week 3:

**53 Anti-Inflammatory Diet Cookbook for Beginners**

## Day 15:

**Breakfast**: Greek yogurt with granola and berries
**Lunch**: Lentil soup with whole-wheat bread
**Dinner**: Chicken stir-fry with broccoli, carrots, and brown rice
**Snack**: Hummus with cucumber slices

## Day 16:

**Breakfast**: Oatmeal with banana and walnuts **Lunch**: Salad with grilled chicken, romaine lettuce,  avocado, and tomato
**Dinner**: Quinoa with grilled Brussels sprouts with salmon
**Snack**: Apple slices with almond butter

## Day 17:

**Breakfast**: Smoothie with spinach, mango, banana, and almond milk
**Lunch**: Leftover chicken stir-fry with broccoli, carrots, and brown rice
**Dinner**: Baked tofu with roasted sweet potatoes and vegetables
**Snack**: Cottage cheese with pineapple and chia seeds

## Day 18:
**54 Anti-Inflammatory Diet Cookbook for Beginners**

**Breakfast**: Onions and bell peppers in scrambled eggs
**Lunch**: avocado and tuna salad sandwich on whole-wheat bread
**Dinner**: Turkey chili with brown rice
**Snack**: Yogurt bark with berries and granola

## Day 19:

**Breakfast**: Greek yogurt with granola and honey
**Lunch**: Quinoa salad with black beans, corn, and avocado
**Dinner**: Salmon with roasted broccoli and brown rice
**Snack**: Apple slices with cinnamon

## Day 20:

**Breakfast**: Berries and chia seeds for overnight oats
**Lunch**: Lentil soup with whole-wheat bread
**Dinner**: Chicken stir-fry with vegetables and brown rice
**Snack**: Nuts, seeds, and dried fruit in trail mix

## Day 21:

**Breakfast**: Smoothie bowl with spinach, banana, mango, and granola
**Lunch**: Leftover chicken stir-fry with vegetables and brown rice

**55 Anti-Inflammatory Diet Cookbook for Beginners**

**Dinner**: roasted sweet potatoes and asparagus paired with baked salmon
**Snack**: Berry-topped Greek yogurt with chia seeds

# Week 4:

## Day 22:

**Breakfast**: Scrambled tofu with spinach and tomatoes
**Lunch**: Quinoa salad with roasted chickpeas, cucumber, and feta cheese
**Dinner**: Lentil soup with whole-wheat bread
**Snack**: Apple slices with peanut butter

## Day 23:

**Breakfast**: Chia seed pudding with coconut milk and fruit
**Lunch**: Chicken salad sandwich on whole-wheat bread with avocado and lettuce
**Dinner**: Turkey burgers on whole-wheat buns with grilled onions and mushrooms
**Snack**: Cottage cheese with pineapple and granola

## Day 24:

**Breakfast**: Overnight oats with chia seeds and nuts
**Lunch**: Salad with grilled salmon, romaine lettuce, quinoa, and avocado
**Dinner**: Vegetarian chili with cornbread
**Snack**: Yogurt bark with berries and granola

## Day 25:

**Breakfast**: Smoothie with spinach, banana, mango, and almond milk
**Lunch:** Leftover lentil soup with whole-wheat bread
**Dinner**: Chicken stir-fry with broccoli, carrots, and brown rice
**Snack**: Hummus with cucumber slices

## Day 26:

**Breakfast**: onions and bell peppers in scrambled eggs
**Lunch**: Turkey chili with brown rice
**Dinner**: quinoa, roasted veggies, and baked tofu
**Snack**: Cottage cheese with pineapple and chia seeds

## Day 27:

**Breakfast**: Greek yogurt with granola and honey
**Lunch**: Chicken Caesar salad with whole-wheat bread

*Dinner*: Salmon with roasted asparagus and quinoa
*Snack*: Dark chocolate and almonds

# Day 28:

**Breakfast**: Overnight oats with berries and nuts **Lunch**: Leftover chicken Caesar salad with whole-wheat bread
**Dinner**: Sweet potato baked with avocado and black beans **Snack**: Edamame

# Day 29:

**Breakfast**: Smoothie with spinach, pineapple, ginger, and almond milk
**Lunch**: Leftover baked sweet potato with black beans and avocado
**Dinner**: Turkey burgers on whole-wheat buns with grilled vegetables
**Snack**: Greek yogurt with granola and honey

# Day 30:

**Breakfast**: Scrambled eggs with smoked salmon and spinach
**Lunch**: grilled chicken and veggies on quinoa salad
**Dinner**: Quinoa with grilled Brussels sprouts with salmon

**58 Anti-Inflammatory Diet Cookbook for Beginners**

**Snack**: Apple slices with almond butter

Congratulations! You have finished the anti-inflammatory meal plan for 30 days. You should now have a better idea of the foods that are beneficial for lowering inflammation and increasing general health. You are free to use this plan as a guideline or to alter it to construct your own antiinflammatory diet. Remember that the key to receiving the advantages of an anti-inflammatory diet is consistency.

# Smart Grocery Shopping for an Anti-Inflammatory Diet

Here are some pointers for anti-inflammatory grocery shopping:

- **Plan your weekly meals and snacks**: This will help you avoid making impulse purchases at the grocery store.
- **Make and stick to a shopping list:** just buy what you need and avoid processed meals.
- **Concentrate on fresh, whole foods:** Fruits, vegetables, whole grains, lean protein, and healthy fats are all good choices.

**59 Anti-Inflammatory Diet Cookbook for Beginners**

- **Carefully read food labels**: Keep an eye out for extra sugars, trans fats, and fake additives.
- **purchase in bulk When possible:** these can save you money and avoid packaging waste.
- **Seasonal produce:** These are often more inexpensive and fresher.
- **Don't be hesitant to explore new foods:** there are many tasty and healthful options.

## Additional Suggestions:

- Whenever possible, get organic produce.
- Grow your own herbs at home.
- Make your meals ahead of time to save time during the week.
- Cook in quantity and store leftovers in the freezer for future meals.

By following these guidelines, you can simply include antiinflammatory concepts into your diet and enjoy tasty, nutritious meals without breaking the bank.

# CHAPTER 9: TIPS FOR LONGTERM SUCCESS

## Incorporating Anti-Inflammatory Habits

Adopting an anti-inflammatory diet is a lifestyle shift rather than a quick remedy. Consider integrating the following habits to ensure long-term success:

**Begin with little steps:** Begin by introducing antiinflammatory items into your current diet. Reduce processed meals, bad fats, and added sugars gradually.

**Plan and cook meals**: Planning ahead of time your meals and snacks will assist you avoid making poor choices when you're hungry. Cook in excess and freeze leftovers for busy days.

**Select anti-inflammatory cooking techniques**: Instead of frying or deep-frying, try grilling, baking, steaming, or poaching.

**Carefully read food labels:** Watch out for hidden sugars, bad fats, and fake additives. Select products that contain simple, whole-food ingredients.

**Concentrate on your entire well-being:** Combine a balanced diet with regular exercise, stress management strategies, and appropriate sleep to improve your overall health and minimize inflammation.

**Rejoice in your accomplishments:** Recognize and appreciate your accomplishments, no matter how minor. You'll be more driven and concentrated as a result.

**Be persistent and patient:** Don't expect immediate results. Making long-term improvements requires time and effort. Recognize your progress and exercise patience with yourself.

## Dealing with Challenges and Setbacks

Everyone faces obstacles and setbacks On their path to a better lifestyle. Here are some pointers for handling them:

**Determine your triggers:** What events or emotions cause you to engage in harmful eating habits? Once you've identified your triggers, you can devise coping strategies to prevent them.

**Be prepared for setbacks:** It is unavoidable that you may make mistakes from time to time. Allow one setback to undermine your entire progress. Get back on track as soon as possible and don't lose up on your goals.

**Be gentle with yourself:** Do not punish yourself for making mistakes. Instead, concentrate on learning from them and moving on.

**Find healthy alternatives:** Find healthier options if you have cravings for harmful meals. For example, instead of ice cream, consider frozen yogurt or a fruit and veggie smoothie.

**Pay attention to progress rather than perfection:** Do not aim for perfection. Instead, focus on moving forward one step at a time. Honor your achievements, no matter how small.

**Remember why you're doing it:** Remind yourself why you embarked on this adventure in the first place. What are your objectives? What do you hope to accomplish? Keeping your goals in mind can assist you in remaining motivated.

**63 Anti-Inflammatory Diet Cookbook for Beginners**

You can successfully adopt an anti-inflammatory diet and experience long-term health advantages by implementing these guidelines. Remember that this is a journey and not a final destination. There will be difficulties along the way, However, with effort and perseverance, you can attain your objectives and achieve ideal health.

# CONCLUSION

## Begin Your Journey to Better Health.

Congratulations on taking the first step toward a more vibrant and healthier you! This anti-inflammatory diet cookbook has given you the knowledge and skills you need to start eating in a new way that prioritizes full, unadulterated foods and reduces inflammation in your body.

Keep in mind that the road to better health is a marathon, not a sprint. Accept the process of learning new recipes, trying new flavors, and discovering your body's unique reactions to different foods. Don't let little blunders discourage you; instead, learn from them and recommit to your goals.

Remember your great potential as you embark on this trip. An anti-inflammatory diet can help you do the following:

- Reduce your chance of developing chronic diseases like heart disease, diabetes, and cancer.
- Improve joint health and pain relief.
- Increase your energy and mood.

**65 Anti-Inflammatory Diet Cookbook for Beginners**

- Improve digestion and intestinal health. Boost your immune system.
- Improve your cognitive function.

Every bite is an opportunity to invest in your health and lay the groundwork for a better future. Accept the pleasure of cooking, the satisfaction of nourishing your body, and the power you have to change your health through the food you eat.

Now, go forth and explore the delectable dishes included within this book, and witness the transformational power of an anti-inflammatory diet. You deserve to live a life full of vigor, energy, and happiness. Take control of your wellbeing and set out on your path.

# INDEX

## ANTI-INFLAMMATORY MEAL PLANNER

DATE: __/__/__

| | Breakfast | Lunch | Dinner | Snacks |
|---|---|---|---|---|
| MON | | | | |
| TUES | | | | |
| WED | | | | |
| THURS | | | | |
| FRI | | | | |
| SAT | | | | |
| SUN | | | | |

# ANTI-INFLAMMATORY MEAL PLANNER

DATE: __/__/__

| | Breakfast | Lunch | Dinner | Snacks |
|---|---|---|---|---|
| MON | | | | |
| TUES | | | | |
| WED | | | | |
| THURS | | | | |
| FRI | | | | |
| SAT | | | | |
| SUN | | | | |

70 Anti-Inflammatory Diet Cookbook for Beginners

# ANTI-INFLAMMATORY MEAL PLANNER

DATE: __/__/__

| | Breakfast | Lunch | Dinner | Snacks |
|---|---|---|---|---|
| MON | | | | |
| TUES | | | | |
| WED | | | | |
| THURS | | | | |
| FRI | | | | |
| SAT | | | | |
| SUN | | | | |

**71 Anti-Inflammatory Diet Cookbook for Beginners**

# ANTI-INFLAMMATORY MEAL PLANNER

DATE: __/__/__

| | Breakfast | Lunch | Dinner | Snacks |
|---|---|---|---|---|
| MON | | | | |
| TUES | | | | |
| WED | | | | |
| THURS | | | | |
| FRI | | | | |
| SAT | | | | |
| SUN | | | | |

72 Anti-Inflammatory Diet Cookbook for Beginners

# ANTI-INFLAMMATORY
## MEAL PLANNER

DATE: __/__/__

| | Breakfast | Lunch | Dinner | Snacks |
|---|---|---|---|---|
| MON | | | | |
| TUES | | | | |
| WED | | | | |
| THURS | | | | |
| FRI | | | | |
| SAT | | | | |
| SUN | | | | |

# ANTI-INFLAMMATORY MEAL PLANNER

DATE: __/__/__

| | Breakfast | Lunch | Dinner | Snacks |
|---|---|---|---|---|
| MON | | | | |
| TUES | | | | |
| WED | | | | |
| THURS | | | | |
| FRI | | | | |
| SAT | | | | |
| SUN | | | | |

74 Anti-Inflammatory Diet Cookbook for Beginners

# ANTI-INFLAMMATORY
# MEAL PLANNER

DATE: __/__/__

| | Breakfast | Lunch | Dinner | Snacks |
|---|---|---|---|---|
| MON | | | | |
| TUES | | | | |
| WED | | | | |
| THURS | | | | |
| FRI | | | | |
| SAT | | | | |
| SUN | | | | |

75 Anti-Inflammatory Diet Cookbook for Beginners

# ANTI-INFLAMMATORY MEAL PLANNER

DATE: __/__/__

| | Breakfast | Lunch | Dinner | Snacks |
|---|---|---|---|---|
| MON | | | | |
| TUES | | | | |
| WED | | | | |
| THURS | | | | |
| FRI | | | | |
| SAT | | | | |
| SUN | | | | |

# ANTI-INFLAMMATORY MEAL PLANNER

DATE: __/__/__

|  | Breakfast | Lunch | Dinner | Snacks |
|---|---|---|---|---|
| MON |  |  |  |  |
| TUES |  |  |  |  |
| WED |  |  |  |  |
| THURS |  |  |  |  |
| FRI |  |  |  |  |
| SAT |  |  |  |  |
| SUN |  |  |  |  |

# ANTI-INFLAMMATORY MEAL PLANNER

DATE: __/__/__

| | Breakfast | Lunch | Dinner | Snacks |
|---|---|---|---|---|
| MON | | | | |
| TUES | | | | |
| WED | | | | |
| THURS | | | | |
| FRI | | | | |
| SAT | | | | |
| SUN | | | | |

# ANTI-INFLAMMATORY MEAL PLANNER

DATE: __/__/__

| | Breakfast | Lunch | Dinner | Snacks |
|---|---|---|---|---|
| **MON** | | | | |
| **TUES** | | | | |
| **WED** | | | | |
| **THURS** | | | | |
| **FRI** | | | | |
| **SAT** | | | | |
| **SUN** | | | | |

# ANTI-INFLAMMATORY MEAL PLANNER

DATE: __/__/__

| | Breakfast | Lunch | Dinner | Snacks |
|---|---|---|---|---|
| MON | | | | |
| TUES | | | | |
| WED | | | | |
| THURS | | | | |
| FRI | | | | |
| SAT | | | | |
| SUN | | | | |

80 Anti-Inflammatory Diet Cookbook for Beginners

# ANTI-INFLAMMATORY MEAL PLANNER

DATE: __/__/__

| | Breakfast | Lunch | Dinner | Snacks |
|---|---|---|---|---|
| **MON** | | | | |
| **TUES** | | | | |
| **WED** | | | | |
| **THURS** | | | | |
| **FRI** | | | | |
| **SAT** | | | | |
| **SUN** | | | | |

**81 Anti-Inflammatory Diet Cookbook for Beginners**

# ANTI-INFLAMMATORY
# MEAL PLANNER

DATE: __/__/__

|  | Breakfast | Lunch | Dinner | Snacks |
|---|---|---|---|---|
| MON |  |  |  |  |
| TUES |  |  |  |  |
| WED |  |  |  |  |
| THURS |  |  |  |  |
| FRI |  |  |  |  |
| SAT |  |  |  |  |
| SUN |  |  |  |  |

# ANTI-INFLAMMATORY MEAL PLANNER

DATE: __/__/__

|  | Breakfast | Lunch | Dinner | Snacks |
|---|---|---|---|---|
| MON |  |  |  |  |
| TUES |  |  |  |  |
| WED |  |  |  |  |
| THURS |  |  |  |  |
| FRI |  |  |  |  |
| SAT |  |  |  |  |
| SUN |  |  |  |  |

# ANTI-INFLAMMATORY
# MEAL PLANNER

DATE: __/__/__

| | Breakfast | Lunch | Dinner | Snacks |
|---|---|---|---|---|
| **MON** | | | | |
| **TUES** | | | | |
| **WED** | | | | |
| **THURS** | | | | |
| **FRI** | | | | |
| **SAT** | | | | |
| **SUN** | | | | |

# ANTI-INFLAMMATORY MEAL PLANNER

DATE: __/__/__

| | Breakfast | Lunch | Dinner | Snacks |
|---|---|---|---|---|
| MON | | | | |
| TUES | | | | |
| WED | | | | |
| THURS | | | | |
| FRI | | | | |
| SAT | | | | |
| SUN | | | | |

**85 Anti-Inflammatory Diet Cookbook for Beginners**

# ANTI-INFLAMMATORY MEAL PLANNER

DATE: __/__/__

| | Breakfast | Lunch | Dinner | Snacks |
|---|---|---|---|---|
| MON | | | | |
| TUES | | | | |
| WED | | | | |
| THURS | | | | |
| FRI | | | | |
| SAT | | | | |
| SUN | | | | |

# ANTI-INFLAMMATORY MEAL PLANNER

DATE: __/__/__

| | Breakfast | Lunch | Dinner | Snacks |
|---|---|---|---|---|
| **MON** | | | | |
| **TUES** | | | | |
| **WED** | | | | |
| **THURS** | | | | |
| **FRI** | | | | |
| **SAT** | | | | |
| **SUN** | | | | |

# ANTI-INFLAMMATORY MEAL PLANNER

DATE: __/__/__

| | Breakfast | Lunch | Dinner | Snacks |
|---|---|---|---|---|
| MON | | | | |
| TUES | | | | |
| WED | | | | |
| THURS | | | | |
| FRI | | | | |
| SAT | | | | |
| SUN | | | | |